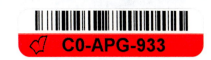

ISBN Paperback: 978-1-64873-547-9

Printed in the United States of America
Published by: Writer's Publishing House
Prescott, AZ 86301

Silent Struggle

Hearing Loss and the Hidden Impact on Mental Health

Doug Dunker ACA, BC-HIS

Board Certified—Hearing Instrument Sciences

American Conference of Audioprosthology

Contents

Preface i

Introduction iii

Chapter 1 Hearing Loss Is Not Just About the Ears 1

Chapter 2 Loneliness in a Room Full of People 9

Chapter 3 Depression, Anxiety, and the Emotional Toll 17

Chapter 4 The Relationship Divide 25

Chapter 5 When the Mind Suffers 33

Chapter 6 Why Hearing Aids Help More Than Your Hearing Loss . 43

Chapter 7 Stories of Change 51

Chapter 8 The Role of Counseling and Support 65

Chapter 9 Tinnitus and the Emotional Spiral 73

Chapter 10 Rethinking Aging, Hearing, and Mental Wellness .. 83

Chapter 11 Building a Better Care Model 91

Chapter 12 You're Not Alone 99

Brain Connections The Science Behind the Stories 105

Appendix A Quick Hearing Self-Check 110

Appendix B Starting the Conversation With a Loved One 111

Appendix C Frequently Asked Questions 112

Appendix D Hearing Appointment Checklist 115

References 120

Prescott Hearing Center and the Author 123

Preface

I've seen it happen more times than I can count.

A person comes into my office thinking they have a memory problem. Or depression. Or anxiety. Sometimes they say they're *"just getting old."* But more often than not, the problem started with something quieter or something they didn't think was a big deal at the time...

Hearing loss.

I'm not referring to a missed word here and there or the occasional misunderstanding. I'm talking about a slow, invisible separation from the world and the emotional weight that comes with it.

Silent Struggle wasn't written to scare you. It was written to be a gentle and honest wake-up call to describe what hearing loss does when it's left untreated. And more importantly, it describes the incredible results that happen when you finally take action.

I've spent years helping people reconnect with their families and themselves by restoring their confidence with better hearing. I've seen laughter return, conversations flow, and strained relationships begin to heal. I've watched parents re-engage with their kids in ways they hadn't in years. I've witnessed expressions

soften and tensions fade from people's faces the moment they begin hearing clearly again. These changes aren't magic, they're what happens when we take hearing loss seriously and treat the whole person and not just the ears.

If you are reading **Silent Struggle**, you already know something is off. You're not broken. You're not crazy. And you're definitely not alone. **Silent Struggle** is for you. Let's take it one page at a time.

Doug Dunker
Prescott Hearing Center

Introduction

What If the Problem Isn't Just Hearing Loss?

Unfortunately, we don't talk about hearing loss the way we talk about other health issues. When someone has high blood pressure, we treat it. When someone is struggling with depression, we try to help. Yet when someone has trouble hearing, we say, *"Eh, that's just part of aging."*

And that's the problem.

Hearing loss is not just a sensory issue. It's not just about turning up the volume or avoiding restaurants. It's a condition that quietly affects your brain, your mood, your relationships, your memory, your identity, and your future.

This book explores the side of hearing loss most people don't talk about - the emotional strain, mental fatigue, and the subtle way it puts pressure on marriages, friendships, and daily life. It's about how confidence and connections slowly erode, not all at once, but through every missed word and misunderstood moment. But most importantly, this book is about what changes when we stop ignoring hearing loss and start taking hearing health seriously.

Inside these chapters, you'll learn:

- Why hearing happens in the brain, not just the ears

- How hearing loss is linked to depression, anxiety, and faster cognitive decline?
- What happens inside the brain when you stop hearing clearly?
- How hearing loss affect families and not just individuals?
- Why treatment, especially early treatment, can help people come back to enjoying a better quality of life?
- What tools, therapies, and support systems really make a difference?
- And most importantly, that you are not alone, and it's not your fault

Whether you're reading this for yourself or for someone you care about, know that you don't have to suffer in silence. You don't have to wait until things get worse to take action. No matter where you are in the journey, it's never too early, or too late, to make a meaningful change.

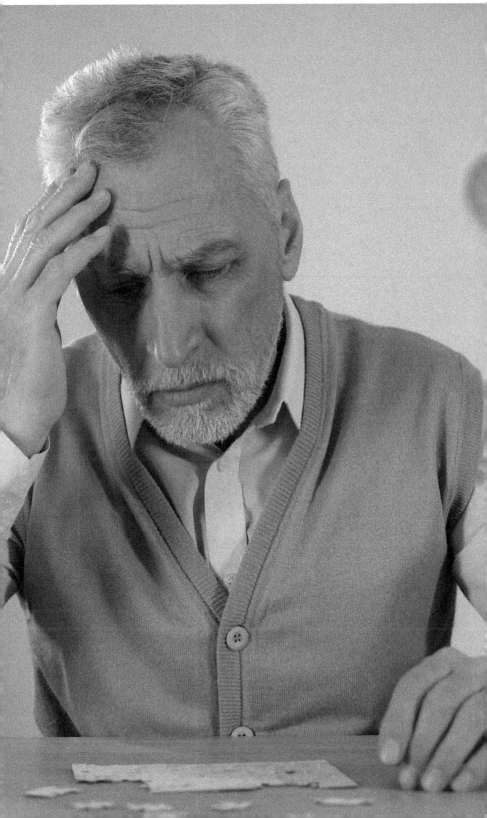

Chapter 1

Hearing Loss Is Not Just About the Ears

Let's start by clearing up one of the biggest misconceptions in healthcare. *Hearing loss is a sensory problem.*

Technically yes, it involves the ears. But in reality, hearing loss is a brain problem with ear-shaped symptoms. The longer hearing loss goes untreated, the more damage it causes - not just to communication, but to cognitive function, emotional stability, and memory. Over time, it can begin to erode a person's sense of identity.

If you've ever looked at someone who is struggling to hear and thought, *"They just need to turn up the volume,"* or *"I need to raise my voice so they can hear me,"* you're missing the point. And frankly, so is much of the medical world.

Your Brain, Not Just Your Ears, Hears

Sound waves hit the ear, but understanding happens in the brain. It's your auditory cortex and its extensive network of collaborators across the brain that turns sound into meaning. And when hearing starts to slip, that entire system is forced to work harder.

You don't just start missing entire words, you start missing parts of words. Your brain is forced to fill in the blanks, guess the meaning, over-analyze the tone, and strain to keep up. That's why people with hearing loss often say they feel mentally exhausted after conversations or group settings. They're not exaggerating.

In fact, a major study out of Johns Hopkins showed that adults with untreated hearing loss had up to 40% faster cognitive decline than their peers. That's not just "being forgetful." That's accelerated brain aging, attributable, in part, to auditory deprivation.

Brain Connection
Deal et al., The Lancet, 2023; Johns Hopkins University
See page 105

Auditory Deprivation: Use It or Lose It

The brain is a use-it-or-lose-it machine. When certain regions go underused, like the ones that process sound and speech, they begin to shrink. That's not a figure of speech, it's measurable. Brain scans show a real loss of gray matter density in people with long-term hearing loss, especially in areas tied to memory, language, and emotional regulation.

Brain Connection
Pronk et al., 2014; Sharma, A.
See page 106

Think about the word *pat*. It's short and simple, but for your brain to understand it, it has to decode three distinct sounds—the "p," the "a," and the crisp "t" at the end. Each sound arrives with its own timing, pitch, and intensity, and the brain pieces them together like a puzzle. If just one sound is missing or unclear, the word becomes meaningless. Is it *pat*? *at*? *sat*? *pass*? The brain is forced to start guessing.

When this happens over and over, the system begins to fray. The auditory cortex doesn't get the signal it needs, so it starts to weaken. The frontal lobe picks up the slack, working overtime to fill in the blanks. Memory systems get overloaded and emotional centers become more reactive. You might feel exhausted after simple conversations, or maybe start withdrawing because social interaction feels like too much work.

This reorganization isn't an efficient process, but rather it is the brain scrambling to compensate. And over time, those changes can lead to cognitive decline. In fact, the Lancet Commission

identified untreated hearing loss as the most common modifiable risk factor for dementia - more than smoking, high blood pressure, or inactivity.

Allow that to sink in...

Brain Connection
Livingston et al., The Lancet, 2020
See page 106

Listening Fatigue: The Invisible Drain

Imagine trying to run your phone on 1% battery all day. That's what listening is like for someone with hearing loss. Every conversation feels like a puzzle, but the pieces are missing or distorted.

This leads to:

- Avoidance of conversations
- Reluctance to join group activities
- A growing sense of isolation and incompetence

Eventually, people stop engaging, not because they don't care, but because their brain is tired. Constantly decoding partial signals

burns through cognitive resources faster than you'd expect. Ironically, the brain is working harder and doing less. That mental drain has consequences.

Compensation Isn't a Long-Term Strategy

People often assume that if they just concentrate harder, they will get by. They start lip-reading, over-analyzing body language, asking *"What?"* more often, or pretending they heard when they don't.

ut compensating is not a long-term strategy. In fact, it eventually backfires. The extra mental work adds stress and distraction, which further impairs memory and focus. And when conversations start to feel like battles, people begin to disengage and the brain gets less stimulation.

Think of it this way. Social interaction is exercise for your brain. When hearing becomes difficult, people stop exercising. We all know what happens to a muscle that doesn't get used.

It's Not Just Age

It's easy to dismiss hearing loss as just a normal part of aging. While it's certainly more common as we get older, that doesn't mean it's harmless. Hearing loss doesn't just affect how you hear,

it influences how your brain functions, how you interact with others, and how you navigate daily life.

What's more concerning is that many people wait seven to ten years after noticing signs of hearing loss before seeking help. That's a long time for the brain to adapt and reorganize in ways that can make things harder in the long run. Unfortunately, the effects aren't always reversible, but they are preventable and treatable.

Early Intervention Is Brain Protection

Here's the good news. Amplifying sound helps restore healthy brain function. When people start using well-fitted hearing aids, the brain regions responsible for sound processing start to re-engage. Cognitive load is reduced and conversations become easier. Social connections increase and with it, mood, memory, and quality of life improve.

This isn't magic. It's biology. And we've seen it in real life, thousands of times.

What's the Takeaway?

- Hearing happens in the brain, not just the ears.
- Untreated hearing loss is linked to cognitive decline, emotional fatigue, and brain shrinkage.

- Early treatment (especially with hearing aids) supports brain health and protects against long-term decline.

If we treated hearing loss like we treat high blood pressure or diabetes, as a legitimate medical issue with real mental health consequences, fewer people would suffer needlessly.

And yet, here we are still asking people if they *"just need to turn it up a bit."* It's time we understood hearing loss for what it is, a whole-brain and whole-life issue. The ears are just the beginning.

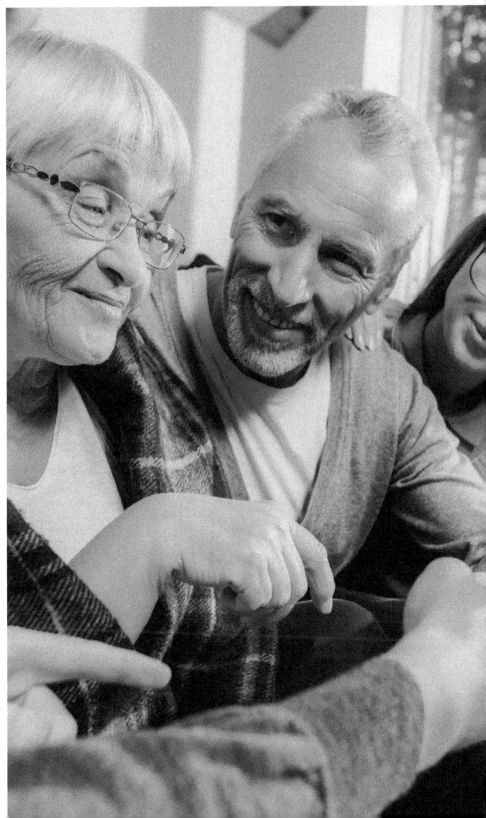

Chapter 2:

Loneliness in a Room Full of People

There's a kind of loneliness that has nothing to do with being alone. It's the feeling of being invisible in a conversation, disconnected in a crowd, or misunderstood at the dinner table. For many people with hearing loss, this is the daily reality of being isolated, not by geography, but by sound.

They are present, but not fully included and engaged. They smile and nod, but don't always catch the joke. And eventually, they stop trying, not because they don't want to connect, but because connections feel out of reach.

This isn't just sad, it's dangerous.

The Social Side of Sound

Human beings are wired for connections. From birth, we learn through voices, tone, laughter, and shared conversation.

Our identities aren't built in isolation but rather take shape through interaction. We define ourselves through conversation, connection, affection, and shared experiences. Storytelling, feedback, laughter, and even disagreement reflect and reinforce

who we are. It's through these moments of engagement that we come to understand our place in the world and how we matter to the people around us.

When hearing begins to slip, people don't just lose access to information, they lose access to interaction. And over time, those missed moments add up.

Think about the grandparent who stops attending family dinners. The spouse who stops participating in group outings. The neighbor who doesn't answer the phone anymore. They don't do these things because they don't care, it's because they're tired of pretending.

The Cost of Withdrawal

Social isolation doesn't just happen like a flip of a switch. It's not a big event that suddenly appears, but rather it creeps in moment by moment. A person might stop going to church, quit volunteering, or neglect chatting with neighbors. They often sit back instead of speaking up and let others talk while they observe from the sidelines.

And somewhere along the line, the narrative changes from *"I didn't hear,"* to *"I don't belong."* This shift is huge. Because once someone internalizes that story, it affects:

- Self-esteem (*"I'm not sharp anymore."*)
- Mood (*"I feel like a burden."*)
- Behavior (*"It's easier to stay home."*)

Studies show that socially isolated adults are at significantly higher risk of depression, anxiety, cognitive decline, and even early mortality. Yes, loneliness, like hearing loss, is a public health threat. And when the two are combined, the effect is amplified.

Brain Connection
National Council on Aging, 1999; Mener et al., 2013
See page 106

The Masking Game

Ask anyone with untreated hearing loss, and they'll tell you that the hardest part is pretending.

They laugh when others laugh, hoping it's not at the wrong time. They bluff through conversations and pray no one notices. They avoid noisy restaurants, crowded rooms, and public events.

All of this takes energy and it creates a difficult paradox. People with hearing loss still want to stay connected and to be part of

conversations and social settings. But being around others can also serve as a painful reminder of how disconnected they've become. So, they begin to pull back, not because they don't care, but because it's exhausting. That withdrawal only deepens the sense of isolation, leading to mood swings, irritability, and quiet resignation. They may insist they're fine, but deep down, they know something's not right.

Loneliness vs. Being Alone

To be clear, being alone is not inherently bad. Solitude can be peaceful and healthy. But loneliness is an involuntary disconnection. It's what happens when someone wants to engage but feels they can't.

In this way, hearing loss creates a form of forced isolation, a sort of invisible barrier between the person and the world around them. One they can't climb over without help.

Worse still, others don't always see what's happening. They may assume:

- *"She's just getting older."*
- *"He's grumpy."*
- *"They don't want to talk."*

And the person with hearing loss feels misunderstood again.

This Doesn't Just Hurt the Individual

Loneliness is contagious. When one person in a social circle disengages, the whole dynamic changes. Family members grow frustrated, friends stop inviting, and spouses stop confiding.

And slowly, relationships that once felt close now feel obligatory and distant.

In some cases, this may lead to:

- Marital strain or resentment
- Caregivers feeling emotionally shut out
- Adult children growing concerned, but unsure how to help

It's not that anyone's trying to disconnect. It's that communication has become too difficult and no one knows how to help.

The Power of Reconnection

The good news is that this pattern doesn't need to be permanent. When hearing loss is identified and treated, especially early, people often experience a noticeable shift. It's not just about hearing more clearly, it's about re-engaging with the world and feeling like yourself again. Clients often say things like, *"I didn't*

realize how much I was missing," or *"I thought I was just depressed,"* or even, *"I feel like I can finally participate again."*

The change doesn't go unnoticed by the people around them either. Conversations become more natural, laughter comes easier, and that spark that had been dimmed by the struggle to keep up starts shining again!

The Takeaway

Hearing loss creates isolation, not just inconvenience. And left untreated, that isolation can erode relationships, self-worth, and mental health. But it's never too late to reconnect.

Helping someone hear again is not just about volume, it's about belonging. It's about making sure no one has to sit silently in a room full of people, wondering what just happened and feeling too embarrassed to ask.

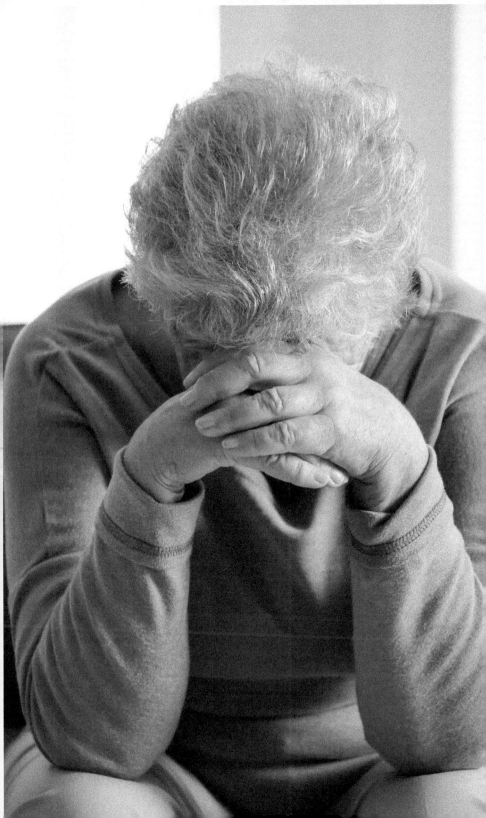

Chapter 3

Depression, Anxiety, and the Emotional Toll

You might expect hearing loss to make life quieter. But in reality, it just makes life feel heavier. Emotionally, socially, and mentally, it takes a toll.

What begins as a minor inconvenience of missing a few words here and there can snowball into something far more destructive. Depression, anxiety, irritability, and hopelessness are commonly the outcome. This is well-documented, and tragically often overlooked.

Still, most people don't connect the dots between hearing and mental health. Unfortunately, many healthcare providers don't bring it up either. That leaves millions of people silently struggling with emotional distress, while not realizing that the root cause is an unaddressed sensory issue dragging their brain and spirit down.

The Emotional Weight of Trying to Keep Up

Imagine starting every conversation a few steps behind. It is like showing up late to a movie and trying to piece together the plot

with half the dialogue missing. You'd feel lost, frustrated, maybe even embarrassed. Multiply that across dozens of conversations every day, and you'll get a sense of what hearing loss does to someone's emotional state.

There's a constant underlying tension and fear:

- *"Did I hear that right?"*
- *"Should I ask them to repeat it again?"*
- *"Did they notice I faked a smile because I missed what they said?"*

This kind of mental gymnastics creates chronic stress, which slowly wears down emotional resilience. It's not only annoying but exhausting too. And when people feel like they're failing at basic communication, their confidence begins to break down. Eventually, they withdraw. Not because they don't want to be involved, but because the effort feels too overwhelming. That's where depression creeps in.

From Frustration to Hopelessness

At first, the emotional response to hearing loss is usually frustration. But left unaddressed, frustration can turn into something deeper and darker.

18

Here's what often happens:

- The person misses key moments in conversations
- They feel embarrassed or ashamed
- They stop participating
- They feel lonely and misunderstood
- They start to believe they no longer matter in the conversation or the relationship

That's the internal progression from inconvenience to isolation and eventually depression.

In fact, studies have shown that older adults with untreated hearing loss are significantly more likely to report symptoms of clinical depression. One major survey reported that older adults with untreated hearing loss were 47% more likely to experience symptoms of depression compared to those who treated their hearing loss.

And it's not just sadness; it's a loss of identity. When people can't express themselves, they start to question who they are. *"I used to be sharp,"* *"I used to be fun,"* and *"Now I just feel like a burden,"* are common themes.

The Constant Threat of Misunderstanding

Where depression shows up as withdrawal, anxiety often shows up as hyper-vigilance. People with hearing loss may become obsessively worried about what they're missing. They overthink conversations, worry about misinterpreting comments, or become afraid of speaking up in case they say something wrong.

It's exhausting to live in that state. Social settings feel like minefields. Phone calls feel like exams. Even casual small talk can trigger anxiety because there's always the possibility of embarrassment.

That's when people start avoiding those situations, not because they're anti-social, but because they're scared of humiliation.

The Family Sees It—But Doesn't Always Understand It

Spouses, children, and close friends often sense that something is off. Their loved one seems more irritable, less engaged, and less joyful. But they may not immediately link it to hearing loss.

That misunderstanding can lead to strained relationships:

- *"Why are you so moody lately?"*
- *"You never want to go anywhere anymore."*
- *"You're not even listening."*

But the truth is, they're trying. And that effort, when it fails, often deepens the emotional wound. This is where empathy becomes essential, not just from professionals, but from loved ones as well.

Untreated Hearing Loss and Suicide Risk

This next part isn't easy to talk about, but it matters. Several studies have found that individuals with hearing loss, particularly younger adults and veterans, face a significantly increased risk of suicidal ideation. The link isn't just theoretical. It's backed by large-scale research from institutions like the NIH and VA.

Brain Connection
Zuelke et al., 2019; U.S. Department of Veterans Affairs, 2019
See page 107

The combination of isolation, frustration, and mental exhaustion can push people into a state of despair. When someone feels like they're fading from the world and no one notices, or worse, no one understands, it's easy to see how hopelessness can take hold. The bottom line is that this is not just an ear issue, it is a life issue.

What Treatment Really Offers

When people finally seek help, are fitted with properly tuned hearing aids, and receive the right support, the change can be

21

remarkable. Conversations become more natural, confidence begins to return, and the constant pressure to pretend or compensate starts to lift. But beyond those functional improvements, many describe something deeper, an emotional relief they didn't expect. They stop feeling broken and start to feel capable again. And for some, that moment marks the first glimpse of light after what felt like a long, quiet tunnel.

The Takeaway

Untreated hearing loss is a slow-motion emotional crisis. It chips away at confidence, fuels depression and anxiety, and leaves people feeling isolated in the very places they most want to belong. Unfortunately, it's not rare, in fact, it's quite common. However, the good news is that it's also treatable.

If we understood the emotional consequences of hearing loss as clearly as we understand the physical ones, far fewer people would suffer in silence. The ears might stop working like they used to. But that doesn't mean life has to be destined for negative emotional changes.

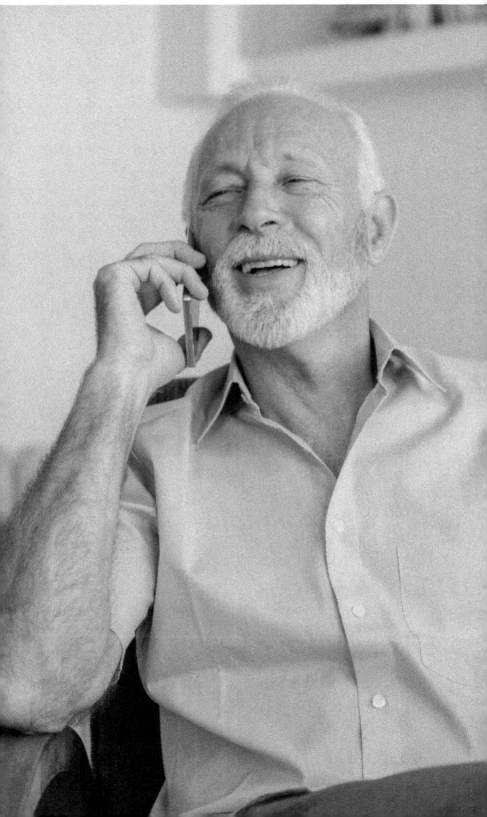

Chapter 4

The Relationship Divide

When hearing starts to go, communication suffers. That part is obvious. What's not always immediately obvious though, is just how deeply it affects relationships.

It starts with a few missed words. Then a few missed moments. Then the entire meaning gets missed. Over time, the emotional tone of a relationship changes, often without anyone realizing the full reason why.

One person feels unheard, while the other feels like a broken record. Conversations grow shorter, more tense, or increasingly one-sided. Resentment builds quietly. The connection begins to erode, and in its place comes silence, not the peaceful kind, but the kind that makes everyone feel alone, even when they're sitting right next to each other.

Chapter Four is about Silence...

Hearing Loss Is a "We" Problem

Here's something that doesn't get said enough: when one person in a relationship has hearing loss, both people live with it.

Whether it's a spouse, sibling, parent, or friend, communication is a two-way street, and when that street becomes hard to navigate, the relationship carries the load.

The hearing partner may grow frustrated from repeating themselves, feel hurt when their loved one seems disengaged, or become embarrassed in social situations when conversations fall apart. Meanwhile, the partner with hearing loss may feel ashamed to admit how much they're missing, defensive when corrected, or left out of jokes, plans, and subtle emotional cues.

Over time, a gap begins to form, not just in conversation, but in emotional closeness, patience, and shared experience.

The Fight That Wasn't About the Dishwasher

In relationships strained by hearing loss, arguments often spark over something small and seemingly insignificant, like what time an appointment was, who forgot to take out the trash, or whether or not the dishwasher was unloaded. *"You never told me we were*

going to the doctor today," "I said it three times," or *"No, you didn't."*

What follows is a familiar tension, frustration, silence, or a full-blown argument. But these fights usually aren't about the appointment, the dishwasher, or the missed detail. They're usually about something deeper - feeling ignored, misunderstood, or emotionally out of sync.

When communication shifts from a source of connection to a source of stress, it opens the door to resentment and emotional distance. That's how hearing loss becomes more than a personal challenge. It becomes a relationship issue.

Emotional Labor and Communication Fatigue

When one partner compensates for the other's hearing loss, it's not just about speaking louder. It's about:

- Adjusting how they talk
- Choosing quieter restaurants
- Taking phone calls on their behalf
- Acting as a translator in group settings

That's called emotional labor, and over time, it gets heavy. Not because they don't love the person, but because they're tired. And

when that fatigue isn't acknowledged, it can lead to frustration or distance that neither person knows how to fix.

On the flip side, the person with hearing loss may feel like a burden. They may start to hold back on sharing thoughts, asking questions, or participating in banter, all to avoid being a hassle.

That self-silencing only deepens the divide.

When Intimacy Changes

Relationships aren't just about words, but they're also about tone, timing, and shared experiences. When hearing loss interrupts those small moments, intimacy suffers.

- A whispered *"I love you"* goes unheard
- A joke is missed and met with confusion instead of laughter
- A moment of vulnerability feels lost when the response is, *"What?"*

Over time, these lapses create emotional distance. Partners may stop confiding. The warmth gets replaced with practical interactions focused around meals, errands, and reminders rather than real conversation.

And in long-term relationships, this shift can feel like grieving a version of the relationship that used to exist.

Family Dynamics and Power Shifts

It's not just romantic partners who are affected. Hearing loss alters dynamics in families too.

Adult children may feel frustrated or worried about aging parents.

- *"Dad never listens anymore."*
- *"Mom won't admit she's struggling."*

Siblings may lose touch because conversations become awkward or too much effort. Friends may stop calling. Grandkids may stop trying to visit on the weekends like they used to.

And if the person with hearing loss is used to being independent or authoritative, needing help with basic communication can feel like a blow to their pride. That often leads to denial, stubbornness, or withdrawal.

Suddenly, the family dynamic is skewed and everyone feels the strain.

Bridging the Divide

The good news is that this doesn't have to be a slow unraveling.

When hearing loss is acknowledged and treated, the tone of a relationship can shift dramatically. Conversations become easier and patience returns. The person with hearing loss feels more confident, and their partner feels less burdened.

But the healing isn't just about hearing aids. It's about learning to communicate differently and together.

That might mean:

- Making eye contact before speaking
- Choosing quiet environments for important conversations
- Being honest about what's heard and what's not
- Addressing emotional tension before it morphs into resentment

In other words, it is learning how to rebuild trust in the conversation.

The Takeaway

Hearing loss puts stress on relationships, not just because of what's missed, but because of how those misses are interpreted as inattention, rejection, or carelessness.

But what's really happening is deeper and more easily fixed. When couples and families face hearing loss together, with compassion and a shared plan, they can turn things around. Not just back to clearer communication, but back to the kind of connections that make relationships worth having in the first place.

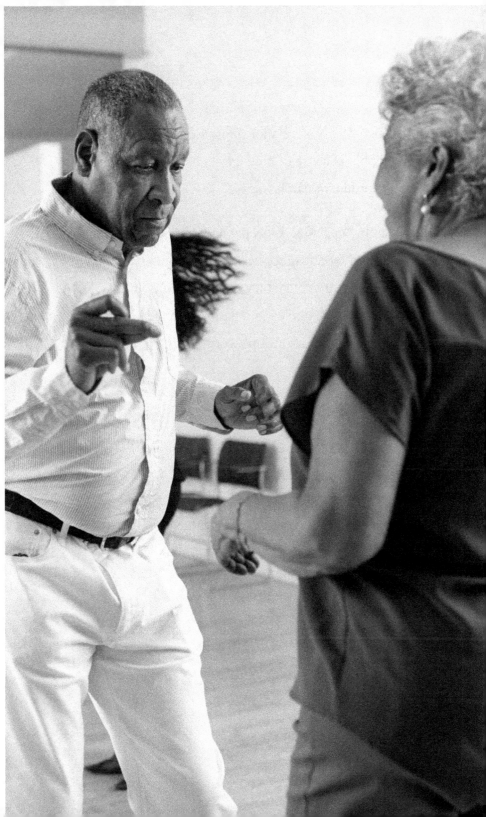

Chapter 5

When the Mind Suffers

If hearing loss only affected the ears, it would be simpler. You'd just crank up the volume and move on with life. But that's not how it works. Hearing doesn't stop at the ear; it continues to the brain.

When the ears stop sending clear signals, the brain doesn't just sit there and wait. It adapts, compensates, and over time, it begins to transform in ways that affect cognition, memory, attention, and even personality.

This isn't science fiction; it's happening quietly, invisibly, and insidiously in millions of people. For many, the signs resemble normal aging and get brushed aside for far too long... until it's too late to reverse the damage.

The Brain Is a Sound Processor

Let's revisit a simple truth. You don't hear with your ears, you hear with your brain.

Sure, your ears collect the sound, but your brain decodes it, figuring out what was said, who said it, what they meant, and how

you should feel about it. It's an enormous amount of work, and it happens in milliseconds.

Now take that stream of sound and start degrading it with garbled words, missing letters and syllables, and distorted volume. The brain has to work harder to make sense of less. That's called cognitive load.

It's the neurological version of "guess and check." And when it becomes constant, it drains resources your brain would normally use for memory, reasoning, and mood regulation.

The Cognitive Toll

Numerous studies have shown a clear link between untreated hearing loss and cognitive decline. The most referenced research comes from Dr. Frank Lin and his team at Johns Hopkins. Over several years, they tracked thousands of older adults and found that those with hearing loss experienced significantly faster rates of cognitive deterioration, including earlier onset of dementia.

Brain Connection
Deal et al., The Lancet, 2023; Johns Hopkins University

See page 105

See page 105

Here's what they found:

- Mild hearing loss doubles the risk of developing dementia
- Moderate hearing loss tripled the risk
- Severe hearing loss increased fivefold

The impact of hearing loss is clear. People with untreated hearing loss scored lower on tests of memory, processing speed, and executive function. In short, the mind suffers when the ears fail.

Brain Shrinkage (Yes, Really)

Here's where things get uncomfortable. Hearing loss is physically linked to brain shrinkage.

MRI scans of older adults with hearing loss show reduced gray matter volume in the auditory cortex, the part of the brain responsible for processing sound. But that's just the beginning. Over time, other areas begin to atrophy too, especially regions involved in memory and language.

Brain Connection
Sharma, A., American Geriatrics Society
See page 108

This is known as auditory deprivation. When the brain no longer receives the sound input it's used to, it begins to redirect resources or let them fade altogether.

Imagine a factory floor where some of the machines suddenly shut down. At first, the remaining machines work overtime to keep production going. But they weren't built to handle the extra load alone, so they start to wear out. Productivity continues to drop. Some departments close entirely. Others take on unfamiliar tasks they're not trained for, leading to confusion and inefficiency. Over time, the factory starts to break down, not just in one area, but across the whole system.

That's what can happen inside the brain when hearing loss is left untreated. It's not just about sound, but it's about what happens when the systems built for processing the sounds are in a forced shut-down mode.

The Domino Effect

Once cognitive function begins to slip, it sets off a chain reaction:

- Memory lapses
- Difficulty concentrating
- Trouble understanding (even with hearing aids later on)
- Loss of independence

People often chalk this up to "normal aging." But hearing loss accelerates these changes. And what's worse, the early warning signs are subtle if not impossible to detect.

A person may seem a little forgetful or distracted. They may start avoiding complex tasks or conversations. Family members might think they're just tired or slowing down. But underneath, the brain is struggling to keep up with a world it no longer hears clearly.

Why the Brain Works So Hard to Compensate

The brain is incredibly adaptive, but it's also a resource hog. When you're missing auditory input, your brain recruits other areas (like the prefrontal cortex) to fill in the blanks. That's why people with hearing loss often feel mentally fatigued at the end of the day.

They're not just "hearing", they're translating, lip-reading, guessing, re-checking, and trying to keep the conversation flowing. That mental energy has to come from somewhere. And often, it comes at the expense of working memory and attention.

This compensation can get people by for a while, but it's like driving a car in low gear. While you can move forward for a while, the strain it places on the engine will undoubtedly cause it to wear out much quicker.

What About People Who Already Show Cognitive Decline?

Another important point is that hearing loss doesn't just increase the risk of dementia; it can complicate the diagnosis.

Why? Because a person with hearing loss might appear more cognitively impaired than they really are. They may not follow instructions, forget what was said, or give inappropriate responses, not because their brain is failing, but because they never heard the question clearly in the first place.

This misinterpretation can lead to:

- Inaccurate dementia diagnoses
- Inappropriate treatment plans
- Missed opportunities for hearing rehabilitation that could improve quality of life

In short, hearing loss can mask, or mimic, cognitive issues. That's why any cognitive screening should always start with a basic hearing assessment.

Can Hearing Aids Help?

Yes, and the research is even more promising.

Recent studies, including the 2023 ACHIEVE trial, show that hearing aid use can slow the rate of cognitive decline, especially

when intervention happens early. People who wear hearing aids consistently show improved performance in verbal memory, executive function, and social engagement compared to those who don't.

Brain Connection
Deal et al., The Lancet, 2023; Johns Hopkins University
See page 105

This isn't to say hearing aids cure dementia, but they give the brain more to work with. They reduce mental fatigue, restore access to communication, and re-engage the parts of the brain that are at risk of going dark.

And in many cases, that's enough to change the trajectory.

The Takeaway

Untreated hearing loss doesn't just make life quieter; it makes life harder. It forces the brain to work overtime, depletes cognitive resources, accelerates aging, and increases the risk of serious neurological decline.

But this isn't inevitable. The earlier hearing loss is identified and treated, the more likely the brain can stay sharp, connected, and resilient. Because in the end, protecting your hearing is protecting your mind.

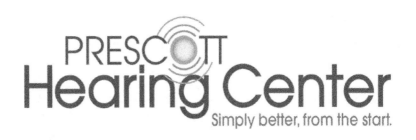

Prescott Hearing Center was established with the goal of providing quality and affordable hearing solutions to the community of Prescott, and the Quad-City area in Yavapai County, Arizona.

Schedule An Appt Now
☎ (928) 899-8104

PrescottHearing.com

Prescott Hearing Center Locations

3108 Clearwater Dr. Suite B2
Prescott, AZ 86305

7762 E. Florentine Rd. Suite D
Prescott Valley, AZ 86314

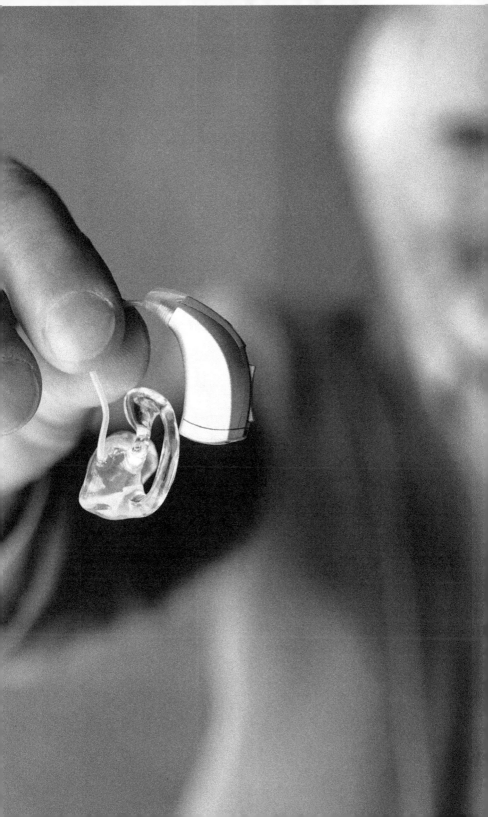

Chapter 6

Why Hearing Aids Help More Than Your Hearing Loss

Most people think of hearing aids as tiny speakers for your ears. They're not wrong. But they're also not quite right either.

Because when used properly, hearing aids don't just help you hear better, they help you live better. They help reconnect people to their families, restore their confidence, enhance their daily routines, enjoy a clever joke, regain their independence, and rediscover joy.

That's not marketing talk. It's the lived experience of millions of people who suffered from hearing loss, and then eventually discovered what they were missing.

Hearing Aids Are Brain Devices (Not Just Ear Devices)

Let's make something clear, the goal of hearing aids isn't to make sound louder, it's to make sound meaningful again.

Remember, hearing happens in the brain. Hearing aids simply help deliver a more complete, balanced, and accurate signal to the auditory cortex. That signal activates underused brain regions,

reduces listening fatigue, and improves your ability to follow conversations in real-time.

Think of hearing aids as rehab for your auditory system. You're not just amplifying; you're retraining your brain to process sound naturally and efficiently.

They Restore Access to Life

One of the cruelest effects of hearing loss is how it robs people of the little things that make life feel rich:

- Hearing your grandchild giggle
- Picking up on your partner's sarcasm
- Catching the punchline without asking, *"Wait, what did he say?"*

Hearing aids put those moments back into play. And when that happens, people light up. They talk more. They smile more. They rejoin conversations instead of fading into the background.

This isn't trivial. This is emotional recovery. You can't treat depression or anxiety in someone with untreated hearing loss without restoring their ability to engage.

They Lower Cognitive Load

We talked in Chapter 5 about the brain's exhausting workaround for missing sound. Hearing aids take care of that struggle.

By improving the clarity and range of incoming sound, they reduce the effort needed to decode speech, especially in challenging environments like restaurants, meetings, or group events. That freed-up brainpower can then go back to doing what it was built for:

- Remembering things
- Processing emotion
- Staying mentally sharp

In other words, hearing aids don't just ease communication, they conserve cognitive fuel.

They Can Slow Down Cognitive Decline

For years, researchers suspected that treating hearing loss might help delay or prevent dementia. Now we have solid data to back it up.

The ACHIEVE study, a major randomized clinical trial published in 2023, found that hearing aid use, combined with proper support, significantly slowed cognitive decline in older adults at risk. This was especially true in people who were already starting

to slip cognitively, the benefits were clear. While hearing aids cannot reverse advanced dementia, they can protect healthy brains from getting there faster. That's prevention in action.

Brain Connection
Deal et al., The Lancet, 2023; Johns Hopkins University
See page 105

They Support Mental Health

Research has shown that treating hearing loss with hearing aids can lead to significant improvements in mental health and overall well-being. Studies have found that individuals who use hearing aids experience fewer symptoms of depression and anxiety, enhanced social confidence, better sleep quality, and greater overall life satisfaction.

Brain Connection
Choi et al., 2020; National Council on Aging, 1999; Mener et al., 2013
See page 108

These benefits highlight that addressing hearing loss is not solely about improving hearing but also about enhancing quality of life across multiple domains. Despite these advantages, many

individuals hesitate to try hearing aids, missing out on the potential for a more connected and fulfilling life.

The Stigma Problem

One of the biggest barriers to hearing aid adoption isn't cost, it's pride. People associate hearing aids with aging, decline, or weakness.

But the irony... What makes someone seem older, weaker, or more out of it?

- Wearing a barely visible hearing aid and engaging fully?
- Constantly mishearing, withdrawing, and checking out?

It really is a simple choice! Today's hearing aids are smarter, sleeker, and more powerful than ever. Many are virtually invisible. Most are Bluetooth-compatible. Some even monitor brain and body health.

This isn't Grandpa's clunky beige banana hanging behind the ear. This is wearable technology that helps you show up for life again.

Why People Wait (and Why They Regret It)

The average person waits seven to ten years between noticing hearing loss and doing something about it. By then, the damage is well underway socially, cognitively, and emotionally.

- So why do they wait so long?
- *"I'm not ready."*
- *"It's not that bad."*
- *"I'll just ask people to repeat."*
- *"I don't want to look old."*
- And what do they say after they finally get hearing aids?
- *"I wish I'd done this years ago."*
- I have never met a hearing aid user that said:
- *"I wish I would have waited a little longer."*

Relearning How to Listen

An important note about hearing aids is that they are not a plug-and-play fix. Hearing aids require:

Adjustment: Your brain needs time to relearn how to interpret amplified sound.

- Fine-tuning: A hearing professional should customize settings for your lifestyle.
- Support: Counseling, follow-ups, and education make all the difference.

This isn't just a hearing device, it's a hearing journey, and the experience is better when you have someone guiding you along the way.

The Takeaway

Hearing aids are far more than electronic devices, they're tools of restoration, dignity, connection, brain health, and of life itself.

They won't make you younger, but they will make you more like yourself again. You'll be more present, confident, and alive.

And if you've been hesitating, don't wait until the silence feels normal. Life is hard enough as it is, you don't need to make it more difficult by trying to cope with hearing loss. You deserve to hear the world, and the people you love, clearly.

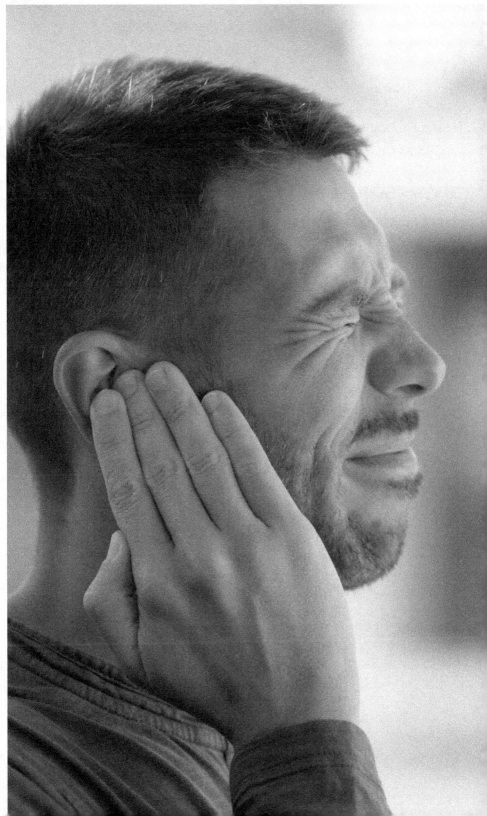

Chapter 7

Stories of Change

Sometimes statistics don't stick. Brain shrinkage, risk multipliers, and cognitive load all matter, but they don't move your heart.

Maybe one of these stories will. Hearing loss isn't just a condition, it's a lived experience and impacts real people with real lives. And when those people finally take action and treat it, something remarkable happens: they come back to life. Sometimes slowly, sometimes like flipping a switch.

This chapter is a reminder that while hearing loss can be isolating, the path back is always within reach.

Tom's Story: "I Thought It Was Just the Ringing"

Tom was frustrated. He was doing everything he could to cope with his tinnitus, but it was wearing him down. The constant noise in his ears was driving him crazy, and he knew it was hurting his quality of life. He struggled to follow conversations at home, at work, and even with the TV on right in front of him. Despite all of that, Tom still believed tinnitus was his real problem.

"If the ringing would just stop," he thought, *"then I'd be able to hear better."*

His doctor didn't help much either. Like many, Tom was told there was nothing he could do for his tinnitus and that he'd just have to learn to live with it. So that's what he did, nothing. It didn't make sense to him to get his hearing checked since the prospect of adding more sound to his world would undoubtedly make things even worse than what he was already experiencing.

But the truth was, it wasn't the tinnitus getting in the way of his hearing, it was the hearing loss feeding the tinnitus. Unfortunately, no one had explained that to him.

When Tom finally came to our office and got properly fitted with hearing aids, everything changed. With sound coming in clearly again, his brain stopped reaching for those phantom noises. His tinnitus had significantly faded into the background. The ringing wasn't gone, but it no longer controlled his day.

For the first time in years, Tom could hear the television without blasting the volume. He could hear his wife in another room. He could follow conversations without feeling lost. And more importantly, he no longer felt helpless.

Tom didn't just get relief from the ringing; he got his life back.

Betty's Story: "I Thought I'd Be Embarrassed"

Betty knew her hearing wasn't what it used to be, but the thought of wearing hearing aids made her cringe. She remembered her mother's devices squealing in public and was embarrassed for her by the unwanted attention and awkward stares. Betty didn't want that for herself. She wasn't ready to feel "old" or answer questions about something she hoped no one would notice. Yet avoiding help came with its own set of embarrassments.

Betty found herself asking people to repeat themselves, sometimes more than once. She'd jump into conversations with responses that didn't make sense, and worse, she knew it. She described it best herself: "When I say something completely off-topic, I feel dumb. It's like I'm not keeping up."

Those moments were starting to add up. She noticed at her work, her church, and even with her family, she felt herself withdrawing in fear of making another mistake. Eventually, this fear of embarrassment from hearing aids became smaller than the embarrassment of going on living without them.

When Betty finally arrived at our office and tried hearing aids, she was stunned. They were so much more discreet than she expected. They were sleek, comfortable, and nearly invisible. But what surprised her most wasn't how they looked; it was how they

sounded. "The clarity," she said, "was like someone turned the lights back on!" She could follow conversations again and didn't need to guess or fake her way through group settings. Her confidence returned and reconnected with others, and felt more like herself again.

Looking back, Betty wishes she'd gotten help sooner. "Now I feel silly that I waited so long. I can't believe I put myself through all those times I spent confused or embarrassed."

Betty didn't just improve her hearing, she got her confidence back, along with her pride.

Joanne's Story: "She Was Still in There"

Ed and his daughter Jennifer brought in Joanne, his wife, and her mom, for a hearing evaluation. The room was quiet and heavy. Joanne had recently been diagnosed with mild cognitive impairment, and the family had already begun grieving the woman they felt they were losing.

Joanne sat in the chair with a distant expression, unsure of her surroundings. When she was addressed, she barely responded. Her family, trying to help, often jumped in to answer for her. "She's just not herself anymore," they said. "She has pretty much checked out."

After the hearing evaluation was performed, Joanne's test revealed a significant hearing loss, with virtually no ability to hear sounds in the speech range. Hearing aids were placed in her ears and we began some small talk. Within moments, everything began to change.

Joanne looked up and responded with clarity, thoughtfulness, and emotion. She wasn't distant anymore as she reconnected with the conversation. The mood in the room shifted. Her family watched in quiet amazement as she began responding with clarity and warmth. Her eyes lit up when she giggled. She was present again.

That day, everything shifted, not just for Joanne, but for Ed and Jennifer, too. What they feared was cognitive decline turned out, in part, to be untreated hearing loss. And while her diagnosis was still real, it was no longer the full picture.

Joanne hadn't simply checked out, she just couldn't hear enough to participate.

Ben's Story: "That's Not What I Heard"

At 43, Ben didn't think much about his hearing. Sure, he'd spent years around noisy equipment, but he still felt young, sharp, and in control. That changed during what should've been a simple evening watching a crime show on television.

The plot of the show was unfolding. The suspect had left a critical piece of evidence at the scene of the crime. The line, *"He left his wife's shoes at the scene of the crime."* Ben was confused. *"Wait, what? Why would he bring his wife's shoes to a crime scene? That doesn't make any sense."*

It wasn't until the trial scene that everything clicked. The prosecutor held up a pair of white tennis shoes. It wasn't the *wife's shoes*, but *white shoes*.

That moment stuck with Ben in a way he didn't expect. It wasn't just a misheard word; it was a complete breakdown of the story. The logic, the connection, and the understanding were all gone. And for Ben, it wasn't funny, it was unsettling.

"I didn't like that feeling," he said. *"That moment where I realized I was completely lost, and I didn't even know why."*

Ben decided he wasn't going to let that happen again and decided to get his hearing tested. He learned that he had high-frequency hearing loss which is common in people with long-term noise exposure. The sounds of speech clarity like *f, s, sh,* and *th*—were already slipping away.

He was fitted with hearing aids, and the difference was immediate. Watching TV was enjoyable again and conversations felt natural. He wasn't guessing anymore.

"I didn't want that cluelessness creeping into other parts of my life," he said. *"That TV show was enough for me."*

Ben didn't wait until things got worse. He took action and stayed connected.

Nikki's Story: "I Didn't Expect Silence"

At just 31, Nikki had been living with tinnitus for nearly two years. The constant ringing was wearing her down both mentally and emotionally. She'd tried to tune it out, but the sound followed her everywhere.

Her hearing test showed only a slight loss, but still technically within the "normal" range of hearing. Even so, she was struggling and not happy with what had happened to her quality of life. Nikki had watched her dad go through something similar. He also had tinnitus, and after years of frustration, found relief through hearing aids. That gave her hope.

She asked to try them. The moment the hearing aids went in, Nikki froze. Then came the tears. For the first time in two years, she experienced complete silence.

It was more than she expected. Not only did the tinnitus disappear, but the world around her sounded clearer and richer. She then connected them to her phone via Bluetooth and was

blown away by the quality of her music. Her favorite podcasts sounded crisp and full, and phone calls were much easier and enjoyable even though she wasn't aware of any significant problem before. "Why doesn't everybody have these?" she exclaimed.

Even better, she no longer had to fumble with bulky earbuds that never seemed to fit. "They'd always pop out or hurt my ears," she said. "These just work."

People sometimes ask if it bothers her to wear hearing aids at such a young age. Nikki just laughs. "Bother me? Not even close. Not when the benefits are this good."

For her, hearing aids weren't a last resort. They were a solution, and a surprisingly powerful one. Nikki didn't wait until things got worse. She took control and got her peace back.

Mary's Story: "It Took Time, But It Was Worth It"

At 78, Mary had been aware of her hearing loss for at least 20 years, probably longer really, if she was honest with herself. She had likely been living with some degree of hearing difficulty for most of her life. But she resisted help, and for decades she had found ways to overcome her challenges by lip reading, smiling and nodding, and avoiding group situations when she could.

When she finally did try hearing devices, they were over-the-counter amplifiers which made everything louder, but not clearer. In a crowd, it was even worse. The poor fit made them uncomfortable and eventually, she gave up. Disappointed and frustrated, she believed hearing aids just wouldn't work for her.

Eventually, her family encouraged her to try again, but this time with professional support. She reluctantly agreed. When she was fitted with real hearing aids, the difference was obvious, but not easy.

If the hearing aids were adjusted appropriately to meet her needs, things sounded strange and unnatural. If they were turned down to where she felt they were comfortable, she couldn't hear clearly. It was a balancing act, and her brain, having been deprived of consistent sound for so long, struggled to adjust.

We explained what was happening, that her auditory system had been working in survival mode, and that her brain needed time to relearn how to make sense of sound. She committed to the process, even though it was frustrating. With ongoing counseling, encouragement, and a lot of patience, Mary didn't give up and kept wearing her hearing aids.

Nearly a year later, something changed. After a routine follow-up visit and a fresh adjustment, she looked up and said, "I can

understand you. It finally sounds… right!" She was surprised when we told her the settings were exactly where they had been on day one. "Then why didn't it work the first time?" she asked.

It wasn't the settings that changed, it was her brain that needed time to catch up. Mary had waited a long time, but in the end, her perseverance gave her what quick fixes never could. Auditory deprivation is a very real condition and its insidious onset makes it nearly impossible to detect. It was Mary's determination and commitment to improvement that allowed her to reconnect with the world again.

She didn't just get used to her hearing aids; she got her world back.

Chapter Summary: The Road Back to Connection

Mary's story reminds us that hearing success doesn't always happen overnight. Sometimes it takes time and may be difficult. But the result is worth it.

When someone says, "Hearing aids don't work," what they often mean is, "It didn't work easily." or "I really didn't want to commit." And for many people, especially those who waited so long, success requires patience, persistence, and a willingness to relearn what the brain has forgotten.

The truth is, the earlier hearing loss is addressed, the smoother the path tends to be. Even when it seems difficult, it's not hopeless. That is actually when it matters most to commit and push through the discomfort, stay consistent, and give yourself a real chance at recovery. The longer hearing loss is left untreated, the harder it can be to reclaim what was lost and unfortunately, the window of opportunity doesn't stay open forever.

I Feel Like Me Again

Believe it or not, the most common phrase we hear from people after they begin treatment is not:

- *"I hear better,"*
- *"It's louder."*
- *"I missed the birds."*
- *The most common phrase is: "I feel like me again."*

Hearing loss doesn't just take away sound. It chips away at laughter, banter, sarcasm, intimacy, curiosity, and everything else that makes you feel like yourself. When people reconnect with better hearing, the emotional lift is unmistakable and quite literally life changing.

Every Story Is a Comeback Story

Look at Tom, Betty, Joanne, Ben, Nikki, and Mary. Each journey started with hesitation or hardship, but every one of them found relief. More importantly, they found their way back to the version of themselves they missed. There's a pattern in all of these stories:

- Denial or delay
- Disconnection or frustration
- A turning point
- Treatment
- Rediscovery and reconnection

And the good news is that the turning point can happen at any time you choose. When someone reconnects and rejoins conversations, laughs at the right moment, and stops pretending to follow along, they're not just hearing again, they're living again.

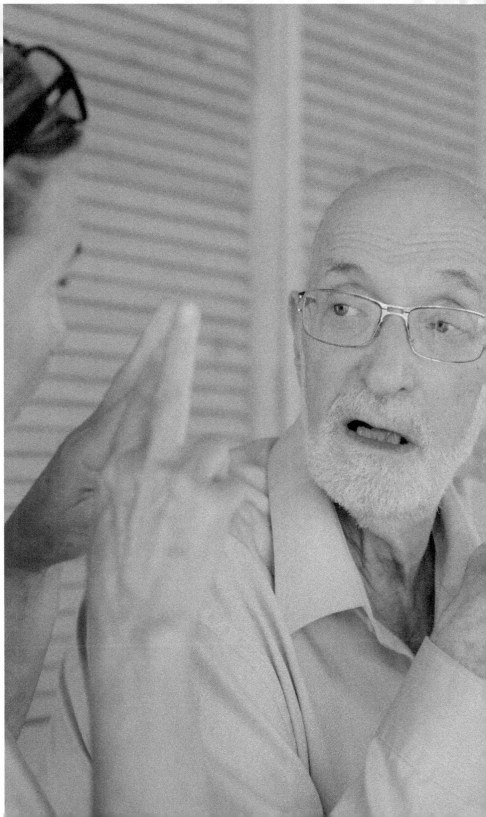

Chapter 8

The Role of Counseling and Support

Fitting hearing aids is science. Helping people live with hearing loss is an art.

You can give someone the most advanced technology on the market, but if they don't feel understood, supported, and empowered, it may never make it out of the case.

That's why hearing care isn't just about the device. It's about the guidance, coaching, reassurances, and honest conversations you have with your hearing healthcare provider. Hearing loss affects more than just the ear canal, it reaches deep into someone's confidence, relationships, and self-image.

If all we do is turn up the volume, we're missing the point.

Why Some People Give Up on Hearing Aids

You've probably heard the line, "I tried hearing aids. They didn't work." But what often happened in those cases is that the user wasn't properly counseled on what to expect, the hearing aids weren't fine-tuned or adjusted over time, and the person may have felt overwhelmed or self-conscious, eventually giving up.

Additionally, no one informed them that it's normal to feel frustrated at first, and there was no one checking in to offer support. We've often heard the line: *"I tried hearing aids. They didn't work."* But here's what actually happened in most of those cases:

- The user wasn't properly counseled on what to expect
- The hearing aids weren't fine-tuned or adjusted over time
- The user felt overwhelmed or self-conscious and gave up
- No one told them it's normal to feel frustrated at first
- There was no one checking in

That's not a failure of technology. That's a failure of support.

Adjustment Is a Process, not a Switch

Getting new hearing aids is like learning to see through new glasses after years of blurry vision, only more complicated. Hearing isn't the same in all situations. It changes with environments, expectations, and emotions.

People often need:

- Time to let their brain adapt to amplified sound
- Counseling to reframe frustrations and normalize setbacks
- Practical tools for handling noisy places, phone calls, or fast talkers

Without that support, it's easy to feel like hearing aids "don't work", when really, they just weren't introduced with enough empathy and clarity.

Communication Strategies Matter

Technology doesn't replace good communication habits. It enhances them. But people still need to learn (or re-learn) how to navigate conversations with hearing loss, both for themselves and with those around them.

This includes:

- Making eye contact before speaking
- Minimizing background noise when possible
- Asking for clarification without shame
- Coaching family members on how to speak clearly instead of loudly

These aren't just tips, they're relationship-saving skills. They often come out of simple counseling sessions where the goal isn't to sell but to listen. Because the real value isn't just in the device, it's in helping someone believe they can thrive with it.

Facing the Emotional Side of Hearing Loss

Let's be honest, hearing loss doesn't just affect your ears. It affects how you feel about yourself, and how you interact with the people around you. Some people feel embarrassed. Others feel old, frustrated, or even broken. They might not say it out loud, but it comes through in hesitation, defensiveness, or jokes that don't feel as funny as they used to.

And for some, the emotional response runs even deeper. Grief is a real part of the journey. It's the quiet realization that something has changed, and might not go back to how it was. That can bring sadness, denial, or even anger. These reactions are completely normal. The important thing is working with someone who understands them, not just clinically, but compassionately.

You're not just looking for a hearing care professional who can only "fix" your hearing, you're looking for someone who walks with you through the transition, gives you the space to process what this change means, and helps you move forward with clarity and confidence.

What to Expect from the Right Provider

The right hearing provider isn't there to sell you a device. They're there to help you reconnect to your relationships, your routines,

your independence, and yourself. This isn't a one-time transaction. It's a guided process.

You want someone who takes the time to understand your goals, not just your audiogram. You need someone who explains things clearly, answers your questions without rushing, and makes sure you feel supported every step of the way. Someone who listens, not just with their ears, but with empathy.

A great provider knows that technology matters, but the relationship matters more. They'll work with you, they'll adjust, and they'll troubleshoot. But most of all, they'll stay committed to helping you succeed.

Hearing Aids Should: Fit Good, Feel Good, and Sound Good

I always tell people that hearing aids need to fit well, feel good, and sound good. All three matter. If one of them is off, you're probably not going to want to wear them. And that's a problem because hearing aids only work when they're actually being used.

That's why the right provider won't just hand you a device and send you on your way. They'll make sure the hearing aids are comfortable in your ears. That the sound quality works for your brain. That the whole experience makes life easier, not more complicated.

Ultimately, wearing hearing aids should feel better than not wearing them. That's the goal, to make communication smoother, connections easier, and daily life more enjoyable. When that happens, the transition becomes something you grow into and enjoy rather than something you fight against.

Support Systems Extend Beyond the Office

Family members, friends, and caregivers also need guidance. Often, they don't know how to help or they unintentionally overhelp, which can come off as condescending.

They may need to learn:

- Patience without being patronizing
- When to repeat something and when to rephrase
- How to encourage without nagging
- How to be a teammate, not a translator
- Because hearing is never a solo sport, but rather a team effort.

The Takeaway

Hearing loss affects more than ears—and so must the solution. Without support, even the best technology can feel frustrating or useless. But with empathy, guidance, and real human connection,

hearing aids become more than a device. They become a bridge back to life.

No one should be handed hearing aids and sent on their way. They should be welcomed into a journey, one that includes their emotions, their relationships, and their hope for what comes next.

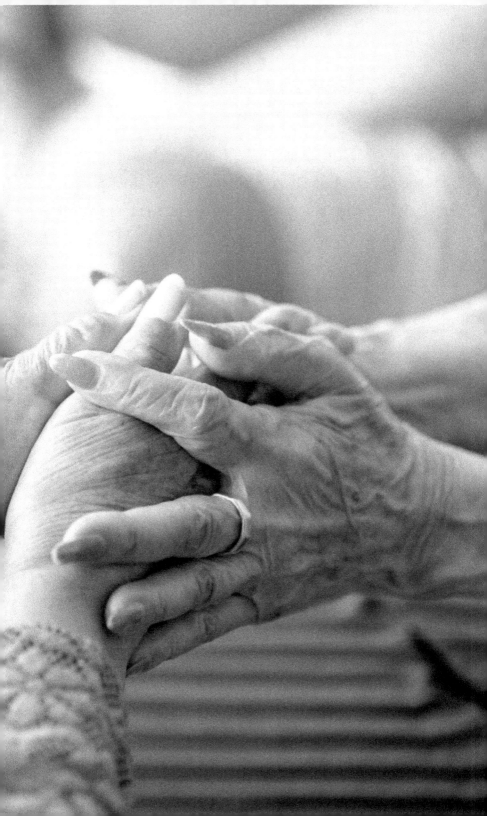

Chapter 9

Tinnitus and the Emotional Spiral

It starts as a faint ringing, maybe only at night. Then it grows. A hum. A buzz. A hiss. A high-pitched tone that won't stop. It's not coming from outside the body. It's coming from within. And worse is that it's invisible. No one else can hear it, no medical procedure can find it, and no single cause can explain it.

Tinnitus is, for many, a slow emotional unraveling. It erodes peace, hijacks sleep, feeds anxiety, and if left untreated, can lead to profound despair and emotional distress.

Let's talk about it. Not just what tinnitus is, but what it does to the brain, your emotions, and to the core being of the people who are trying to live with it.

What Is Tinnitus, Really?

Tinnitus is the perception of sound when no external sound is present. That part is simple. What's not so simple is everything else:

- It may be constant or intermittent
- It may be high-pitched, pulsing, clicking, hissing, roaring

- It may affect one ear or both
- It may come from hearing loss, noise exposure, head trauma, medication, stress, or seemingly nothing at all.

And that uncertainty makes everything seem worse. Because now, in addition to the sound, you have fear.

- *"What's causing this?"*
- *"Will it get worse?"*
- *"Is it going to drive me crazy?"*

For some people, it's a mild annoyance, and for others, it's an invisible tormentor.

The Brain's Role in the Noise

While the ear may be triggering the sound, it's the brain that creates the experience. Tinnitus is often the brain's overreaction to missing input from the auditory system. When the ears stop sending full signals (as with hearing loss), the brain turns up its internal gain. It tries to "listen harder," and in that process, it begins to generate phantom noise.

Brain Connection
American Tinnitus Association; Jastreboff, P. J.
See page 109

It's like a microphone feeding back when it can't find a signal. Except this microphone is in your head. And this is where things get even trickier. Once the brain starts focusing on the sound, it pulls in help from other parts of the brain, particularly the limbic system, which processes emotions, and the autonomic nervous system, which controls stress and arousal. That's how a sound that started as harmless becomes perceived as a threat.

Brain Connection
Cleveland Clinic
See page 109

The Emotional Spiral Begins

When tinnitus becomes bothersome, the brain starts to associate it with danger. Even if you rationally know it won't hurt you, your body disagrees.

You feel:

- Anxious
- On edge
- Irritable
- Distracted
- Exhausted

And that reaction creates more stress which makes the tinnitus feel louder, which in turn creates more stress. As the feedback loop builds, the negative emotions spiral. Now you're not just hearing the noise, you're afraid of it, and the fight begins to try and eliminate it.

Sleep and Sanity

Tinnitus often seems to get worse at night. It's not because it's louder, but because the world is quieter. Since there are no distractions or background noise, all you hear is the ringing.

That leads to:

- Delayed sleep onset
- Poor sleep quality
- Night-time anxiety
- Fear of going to bed

And as we know, sleep loss impairs mood regulation, concentration, and overall resilience. The next day becomes harder, the tinnitus seems worse, and the cycle continues. This is how people with severe tinnitus often end up with depression, anxiety disorders, and panic attacks. Not because they're mentally fragile, but because the brain doesn't do well under constant, inescapable stimuli with no control or resolution.

The Isolation Factor

What makes tinnitus especially cruel is that no one else hears it. There's no bleeding, no swelling, no visible sign that anything's wrong. On the outside, you look fine, but inside, it's a different story. That disconnect can leave people feeling profoundly alone.

They stop talking about it because others don't understand. They worry about being dismissed with comments like, *"It's just a little ringing - just ignore it."* Over time, they begin to doubt their own resilience. They wonder if it will ever stop and fear that it won't.

That sense of isolation, layered on top of the sound itself, turns tinnitus into a mental health crisis hiding in plain sight.

So What Actually Helps?

First, let's start with the bad news - there's no universal cure.

Now the good news - there is relief!

For many people, the relief is life-changing. Most successful tinnitus management falls into one of the following three main categories.

Sound Therapy and Hearing Aids

When tinnitus is linked to hearing loss, properly fitted hearing aids can be a highly effective treatment. By restoring ambient sound and stimulating the auditory system, they:

- Provide appropriate gain where hearing is diminished
- Reduce the brain's gain response
- Cover or mask the tinnitus
- Give the brain something real to listen to

Many hearing aids also include built-in sound generators like ocean waves, white noise, or nature sounds, designed to shift attention away from the ringing. For many patients, this alone reduces their tinnitus perception significantly.

And even when hearing loss isn't severe, mild amplification can improve the brain's input enough to dampen the overactivity driving tinnitus.

Cognitive-behavioral therapy (CBT)

CBT is the gold standard for addressing the emotional side of tinnitus. It helps patients:

- Reframe negative beliefs (*"This is ruining my life"* becomes *"This is annoying but manageable."*)

- Reduce catastrophic thinking
- Learn coping strategies and relaxation techniques
- Break the anxiety-tinnitus feedback loop

CBT doesn't make the sound disappear, but it makes it less scary, less intrusive, and less important. For most sufferers, that's a game-changer.

Tinnitus Retraining Therapy (TRT) and Habituation

TRT combines sound therapy with counseling to help the brain learn to tune out the tinnitus signal. Just like you ignore the feeling of your clothes or the hum of a refrigerator.

This process, called habituation, takes time. But when it works, people often report they don't really notice the tinnitus anymore. It's not gone. But it no longer dominates their life.

Other Supportive Tools

- While not primary treatments, the following may also help manage tinnitus-related distress:
- Meditation and mindfulness (to reduce reactivity)
- Sleep aids or routines (to protect rest)
- Exercise (to regulate stress hormones)
- Support groups (to break isolation)

Nutrition and hydration (some report sensitivity to caffeine, alcohol, or high-salt diets)

Every person's journey is different. The key is knowing there is help in finding options. Once they do, the spiral starts to reverse.

Finding the Right Support

If you're struggling with tinnitus or watching someone you care about suffer from it, you've probably heard the phrase, *"There's nothing you can do."* Maybe from a doctor, maybe from a friend, maybe even from yourself. But that's not the full story.

Tinnitus may not be curable, but it is treatable. And the first step is finding someone who actually listens. You want a provider who won't brush it off or rush through the appointment. Someone who can explain what's happening in your brain in a way that makes sense. Someone who offers realistic options, not empty promises. Someone who doesn't just hand you a device, but walks with you through the process, step by step. Hope is real, and with the right support, relief is possible.

The Takeaway

Tinnitus is more than a sound. It's an experience that affects the brain, the body, and the heart. And for some, it's the most

emotionally taxing part of hearing loss. It doesn't have to stay that way.

With the right tools, education, and support, people can reclaim peace. Not by silencing the noise, but by turning down its power. When that happens, they don't just get relief, they get their lives back.

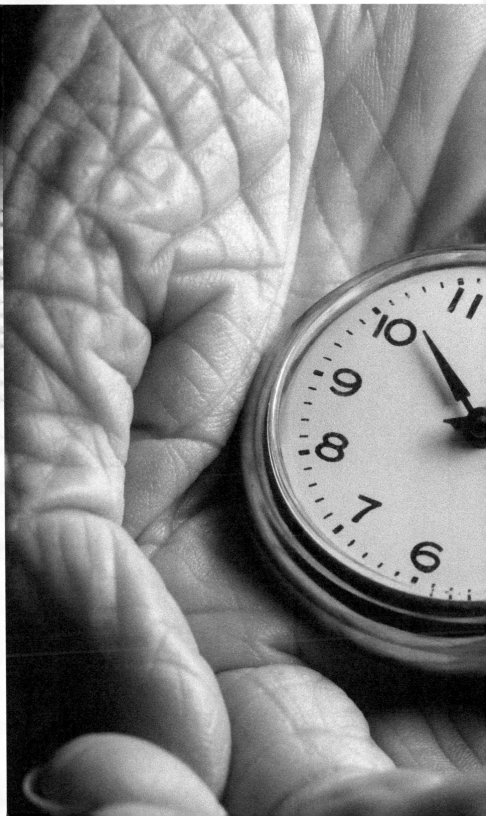

Chapter 10

Rethinking Aging, Hearing, and Mental Wellness

We've been fed a myth.

- That hearing loss is just *"part of getting old"*
- That it's no big deal
- That it's inevitable, unfixable, and not worth worrying about

And that myth has cost us dearly because it convinces people to wait. It suggests that we simply dismiss the early signs and make the best of a bad situation. We should quietly slip into isolation and decline while brushing it off as "just aging."

Let's be clear, getting older doesn't have to mean getting disconnected. But first, we have to change the way we talk about aging, hearing, and mental wellness, not just in the hearing care world, but in our culture at large.

The False Equation: Hearing Loss = Old Age = Decline

Many people see hearing loss as a marker of decline. Like gray hair or slower steps, they treat it as a symbol that their best years are behind them. That's why so many resist hearing aids, not

because they don't want to hear better, but because they don't want to feel "old."

But here's the irony; ignoring hearing loss is what accelerates aging.

- It drains the brain
- It shrinks social circles
- It feeds depression
- It speeds cognitive decline

If anything, treating hearing loss is one of the most age-defying things a person can do. It preserves independence, keeps the mind sharp, and lets people stay connected to the world around them. That's not "getting old." That's staying engaged.

Normalizing Help Without Stigma

No one blinks an eye when someone puts on glasses. Nobody says, *"Oh wow, you wear glasses? That's too bad, you must be falling apart."* But when it comes to hearing aids, people hesitate. Why? Because hearing loss is still wrongly associated with aging, frailty, or decline.

It's time to let that go.

Modern hearing devices are sleek, smart, and often nearly invisible. Many even connect via Bluetooth, allowing you to take

phone calls, stream music, or listen to podcasts and videos directly through your hearing aids, turning them into wireless earbuds with enviable benefits.

But more importantly, they're empowering. They help people keep doing the things that matter most including having conversations, attending events, working, traveling, volunteering, and staying active with their families and communities.

If we start viewing hearing support like we view a fitness tracker, a quality chair, or a great pair of shoes, as tools that help us function at our best, then hearing aids stop looking like a sign of loss and start looking like a healthy upgrade.

Mental Health Isn't a Side Effect - It's the Core

There's also a long-overdue shift happening in how we think about mental wellness in aging. For decades, older adults have been expected to just "deal with" their sadness, confusion, or withdrawal. *"It's just part of getting older,"* people say. But that's lazy thinking and it's wrong.

Many of the mental health challenges older adults face are preventable. Hearing loss is one of the biggest levers we can pull to prevent those challenges.

What if:

- Depression in older adults was routinely screened with hearing.

- Memory complaints triggered both cognitive and hearing evaluations.

- Loneliness was recognized not as a personality trait, but as a sensory-access issue.

We'd catch more problems earlier. We'd treat them more holistically. And we'd help more people stay well, not just longer, but better.

The Longevity Gap vs. the Vitality Gap

We've made great progress in extending human life. But we haven't done as well in lengthening human vitality. Too many people spend their later years disconnected, confused, isolated, and resigned when they could be:

- Traveling
- Learning
- Contributing
- Laughing
- Mentoring

And yes, hearing plays a massive role in all of that. If you can't participate in a conversation, your world shrinks. But when you hear clearly, your world opens up. And with it comes confidence, curiosity, and emotional resilience. That's not just aging gracefully, that's aging boldly.

What to Look for in a Provider

The right hearing provider isn't just there to treat your ears, they're there to protect your quality of life. That mindset makes a big difference.

A great provider will ask about more than just your hearing test. They'll check in on your mood, your mental health, and how hearing loss is affecting your relationships. They'll take the time to understand your fears and frustrations, and they won't brush them off. If needed, they'll coordinate with other professionals, like mental health providers to give you the support you deserve.

This isn't just about devices, it's about dignity. When hearing loss is treated early and thoroughly, it's not just your hearing that improves. It's your ability to stay connected, engaged, and fully present in the life you want to live.

A New Narrative

Here's what we want people to believe and feel about hearing and aging:

- Getting older doesn't mean fading out
- Asking for help is a sign of strength
- Hearing loss is common, but so is treatment
- Staying connected is one of the best things you can do for your brain

It's never too early, or too late, to take action

This isn't about sugar-coating the reality of aging. It's about reclaiming the power that comes with staying engaged. And hearing is one of the most powerful tools we have.

The Takeaway

Aging doesn't mean disappearing and hearing loss doesn't mean decline. And treating hearing loss isn't giving in, it's showing up.

It's time to ditch the stigma, rewrite the assumptions, and make sure people understand that good hearing health is one of the most important investments they can make for their mind, their mood, and their future.

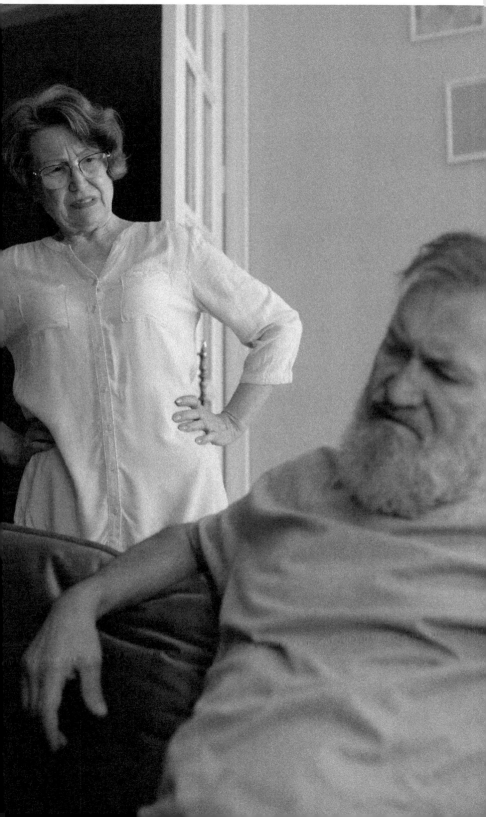

Chapter 11

Building a Better Care Model

If hearing loss impacts nearly half of adults over 60 and is linked to cognitive decline, depression, physical falls, social isolation, and dementia, why doesn't it receive the attention of a critical health concern?

The simple answer is that we haven't built the right care model.

Hearing care often exists on the fringe of medicine. It's rarely integrated, poorly reimbursed, and inconsistently screened. As a result, millions of people fall through the cracks, not because help doesn't exist, but because the healthcare system often overlooks the role of hearing in communication, early intervention, and emotional well-being.

This chapter isn't a rant. It's a call to action. Because the opportunity is right in front of us.

The Current Model: Fragmented and Failing

Here's what typically happens:

- A patient complains of memory problems
- They're referred to neurology or psychiatry

- No one asks about their hearing
- If they do, they're told *"It's just age"* or handed a brochure
- Years pass and the brain compensates, then declines
- They arrive at audiology with frustration, fatigue, and fear

By the time most hearing loss is treated, the emotional and cognitive effects have already taken hold. In some cases, the delay makes it harder for the brain to adjust to hearing aids at all, making treatment less effective than it could have been.

This reactive model isn't working. What we need is a proactive, integrated approach, one that treats hearing as the vital health function it truly is.

Where We Break Down

Let's look at the major system failures:

1. Lack of Routine Hearing Screening

Most adults over 50 are never screened for hearing unless they complain. Even then, it's often minimized. Compare that to blood pressure, cholesterol, and glucose which are routinely tested regardless of symptoms. We need to make hearing screening a standard part of adult wellness care.

2. Poor Integration with Primary Care

Primary care providers are often the first to hear complaints about isolation, forgetfulness, or mood swings, but rarely connect them to hearing loss. This isn't neglect, it's a training gap. Medical schools spend very little time on auditory health. As a result, primary care remains disconnected from hearing care, although early intervention could prevent many downstream issues.

3. Insurance and Access Barriers

In many healthcare systems, hearing aids and hearing care aren't covered or are only partially reimbursed. This sends a clear (and dangerous) message that "hearing isn't essential." But if hearing loss increases fall risk, worsens mental health, and raises dementia risk, how is it not essential? The system needs to catch up with the research.

The Mental Health Disconnect

Mental health providers frequently see clients with:

- Anxiety
- Depression
- Sleep disturbances
- Social withdrawal
- Cognitive complaints

Many of these symptoms can be compounded or even caused by untreated hearing loss.

And yet?

- Most mental health professionals aren't trained to screen for hearing loss
- Most hearing care professionals aren't trained to address emotional health
- Patients are left bouncing between providers with no one connecting the dots

Hearing care and mental health care must be aligned for shared strategies and responsibility.

A Better Model Is Possible

What would a truly integrated hearing care model look like?

1. **Routine Screening & Education**
   - Hearing screenings included in annual physicals starting at age 50
   - Patient education on how hearing affects brain and emotional health
   - Clear referral pathways between primary care and hearing clinics

2. Whole-Person Hearing Care

- Hearing care professionals trained to recognize and support emotional health
- Counseling built into hearing aid fittings
- Collaboration with mental health professionals when needed

3. Team-Based Care

- Primary care, hearing care, mental health, and geriatrics working together
- Shared records, care plans, and accountability
- Patient-centered language focused on outcomes, not devices

4. Policy Change

- Insurance coverage that treats hearing care as medically necessary
- Medicare expansion to cover hearing aids and counseling
- Public health messaging that frames hearing loss as a preventable risk and not just a nuisance

5. Technology with Support

- Yes, over-the-counter hearing aids are a step toward access
- But without counseling, customization, and follow-up, many users will fail
- Technology must be paired with human support to deliver true outcomes

The Role of Advocacy and Awareness

Professionals can only do so much within a broken system. What's needed now is pressure from patients, providers, and the public to elevate the conversation.

- Advocacy for insurance reform
- Public education campaigns
- Interdisciplinary conferences and research
- Media stories that humanize the impact of hearing loss

We don't need another study showing the link between hearing loss and mental decline. We need action.

The Takeaway

The current system treats hearing loss as optional, hearing aids as elective, and hearing care as niche. But the data tells a different

story. Hearing loss is a gateway issue to isolation, decline, and suffering. Treating it early isn't a luxury, but rather preventative medicine.

We have the tools and the science. Now we need a model that brings it all together and treats people as if their ability to connect, think, and hear clearly actually matters.

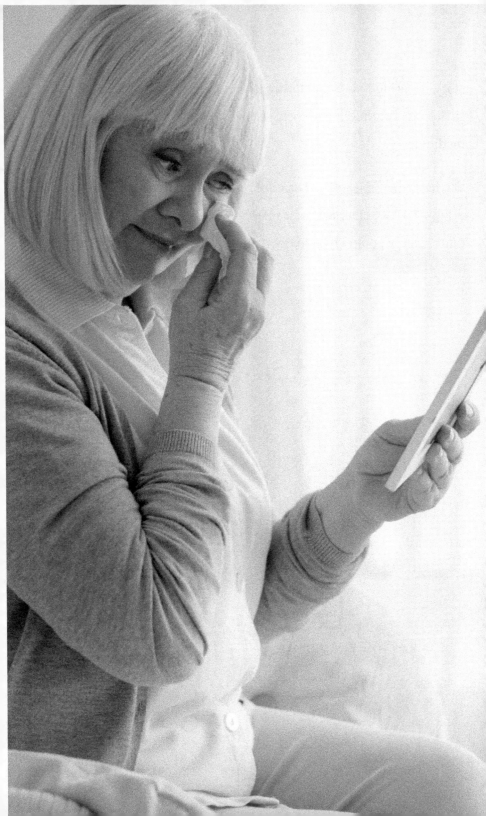

Chapter 12

You're Not Alone

If you've made it this far, you've probably recognized something important:

Hearing loss isn't just about sound. It's about identity, relationships, emotional health, brain function, and everyday life. It's personal. It's real. And for millions of people, it's hidden in shame or denial.

So, let's be clear and direct when we say:

- You're not imagining things
- You're not being "too sensitive."
- And you're definitely not alone.

This Struggle Is More Common Than You Think

Hearing loss affects more people than you realize:

- Nearly 1 in 3 adults over age 65.
- 1 in 2 over age 75.
- Millions more are younger, including veterans, musicians, tech workers, and people who've simply lived noisy lives.

And yet, so many feel alone and isolated in their experience because the symptoms are invisible, the emotions are complex, and the path to help can feel uncertain. You are not broken. You are not weak. You are dealing with something real and you don't have to do it in silence.

You Don't Have to Wait Until It Gets Worse

Most people don't treat hearing loss when it begins. They wait until it interferes with family, social life, memory, or mood. They wait until the damage shows up somewhere else and then they rush to fix a bigger problem. By now you know that it doesn't have to be that way.

Early action means:

- Better results
- Less strain on your brain
- More time spent engaged in the life you've built

Even if it feels small now and even if you miss just a few words or ask people to repeat themselves, it's worth getting it checked out. The cost of waiting is higher than the cost of early treatment. The cost of waiting is higher than most people ever realize.

There Is Help and It Works.

Today's hearing care is not what it used to be. It's smarter, more personalized, more compassionate, and far more effective than most people expect. The best providers don't just hand you a device; they walk you through every step of the way, helping you navigate the frustrations, the doubts, and the hope.

And the tools are powerful. Modern hearing aids can connect to your phone, stream music, enhance speech in noise, and deliver sounds your brain forgot how to hear. But more importantly, they reconnect you to people, to purpose, and yourself.

You Still Get to Be You

Hearing loss doesn't erase who you are. In fact, most people who begin treatment say *"I feel like myself again."* You're not just hearing birds or beeps, you're hearing your spouse's laugh, your best friend's sarcasm, or your grandchild's first words. You're hearing life again. That spark you thought you lost is still there. It's just been waiting to be heard.

If You're Supporting Someone Else

If you're reading this as a loved one, know that your support matters more than you realize.

- Your patience helps rebuild confidence
- Your encouragement may be the nudge they need
- Your presence makes them feel less alone in the process

You don't need to be perfect, just be present.

And when the moment comes to talk about hearing care, make it about life and not just loss. Ask what they miss. Ask what they want to feel like again. Because that's what treatment can give back.

Let's End with This

Hearing loss is real, and its effects can reach into every part of life. But it doesn't have to define your future. There are solutions. There is support. There are trained and compassionate people committed to helping you reconnect with the world around you. But most importantly, there is hope.

Whether your struggle is subtle or overwhelming, recent or lifelong, you don't have to face it alone. And with the right help, a better life is within your reach.

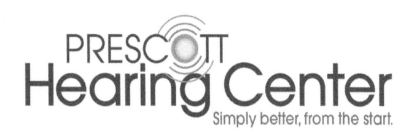

PRESCOTT Hearing Center

Simply better, from the start.

Prescott Hearing Center was established with the goal of providing quality and affordable hearing solutions to the community of Prescott, and the Quad-City area in Yavapai County, Arizona.

Schedule An Appt Now
☎ (928) 899-8104

PrescottHearing.com

Prescott Hearing Center Locations

3108 Clearwater Dr. Suite B2
Prescott, AZ 86305

7762 E. Florentine Rd. Suite D
Prescott Valley, AZ 86314

Brain Connections

The Science Behind the Stories

These science callouts appear throughout the book. Below you'll find a deeper dive into each subject, along with the chapter where it appears.

 Johns Hopkins & The ACHIEVE Study: Hearing and Cognitive Health

Appears in Chapter 1 - "Your Brain, Not Just Your Ears, Hears"

Appears in Chapter 5 - "The Cognitive Toll"

Appears in Chapter 5 - "Can Hearing Aids Help?"

Appears in Chapter 6 - "They Can Slow Down Cognitive Decline"

Pioneering research from Johns Hopkins University, led by Dr. Frank Lin, has demonstrated a clear link between untreated hearing loss and accelerated cognitive decline. Their large-scale ACHIEVE trial (2023) confirmed that treating hearing loss in at-risk older adults helped slow cognitive decline—marking one of the first controlled studies to do so. The takeaway? Treating hearing loss is not just about sound. It's about protecting your brain.

Source: *Deal et al., The Lancet, 2023; Johns Hopkins University*

Auditory Deprivation and Brain Rewiring

Appears in Chapter 1 - "Auditory Deprivation: Use It or Lose It"

When hearing loss goes untreated, the brain receives less stimulation in the auditory regions. This lack of input, called auditory deprivation, can cause the brain to weaken or reroute the pathways responsible for understanding speech. That's why adapting to hearing aids can take time: the brain has to relearn how to hear.
***Source:** Pronk et al., 2014; Sharma, A.*

 Hearing Loss and Dementia Risk

Appears in Chapter 1 - Auditory Deprivation: Use It or Lose It"

The Lancet Commission (2020) identified untreated hearing loss as the #1 most significant modifiable risk factor for dementia, surpassing smoking, hypertension, and inactivity. Addressing hearing loss early not only improves daily communication but may also reduce long-term cognitive decline.
***Source:** Livingston et al., The Lancet, 2020*

 Emotional Distress and Hearing Loss

Appears in Chapter 2 - "The Cost of Withdrawal"

People with untreated hearing loss are significantly more likely to experience depression, social isolation, and emotional fatigue. A major study from the National Council on Aging found that older adults with untreated hearing loss were 47% more likely to report depressive symptoms. Emotional well-being is closely tied to our ability to communicate and connect.

Source: *National Council on Aging, 1999; Mener et al., 2013*

Suicide Risk and Hearing Loss

Appears in Chapter 3 - "Untreated Hearing Loss and Suicide Risk"

Data from the NIH and Department of Veterans Affairs shows a higher risk of suicidal thoughts in people with hearing loss, especially among younger adults and veterans. While hearing loss doesn't directly cause suicidal ideation, it can intensify feelings of isolation, anxiety, and helplessness, particularly when left untreated.

Sources: *Zuelke et al., 2019; U.S. Department of Veterans Affairs, 2019*

Brain Shrinkage and Untreated Hearing Loss

Appears in Chapter 5 - "Brain Shrinkage (Yes, Really)"

Research led by Dr. Anu Sharma has shown that untreated hearing loss can result in reduced gray matter in the auditory cortex. This happens because the brain is highly adaptive and if it isn't receiving sound input, it reallocates those regions for other functions. Over time, this "reassignment" may compromise memory, attention, and language processing.

Source: *Sharma, A., American Geriatrics Society*

 Hearing Aids and Quality of Life

Appears in Chapter 6 - "They Support Mental Health"

Research shows that hearing aids not only improve communication but also significantly enhance overall quality of life. Users report reduced symptoms of depression, less anxiety, decreased social isolation, and improved relationships. Hearing aids help people stay active, feel more confident, and re-engage with the world around them—benefits that reach far beyond the ears.

Sources: *Choi et al., 2020; National Council on Aging, 1999; Mener et al., 2013*

Tinnitus and the Brain's Hyperactivity

Appears in Chapter 9 - "The Brain's Role in the Noise"

Tinnitus often originates from hearing loss, but it's sustained by the brain. When auditory input is reduced, the brain increases its internal "gain," or sensitivity to sound. This overcompensation may result in the perception of phantom noise. Functional imaging shows hyperactivity in both the auditory cortex and limbic system, which explains why tinnitus can feel both persistent and emotionally draining.
Source: *American Tinnitus Association; Jastreboff, P. J.*

 The Limbic System and Emotional Response

Appears in Chapter 9 - "The Brain's Role in the Noise"

The limbic system is a set of brain structures that play a key role in processing emotions, behavior, motivation, and memory. When hearing becomes difficult, the brain leans more heavily on this system to make sense of communication. This added burden can lead to increased irritability, emotional fatigue, and even social withdrawal. The constant strain of trying to interpret incomplete sound can make everyday interactions feel overwhelming.
Source: *Cleveland Clinic*

Appendix A

Quick Hearing Self-Check

Not sure if you or someone you love has hearing loss? Start here.

Ask yourself: Do you...

- Strain to follow conversations in restaurants or groups?
- Are women and children hard to understand?
- Often ask people to repeat themselves.
- Feel like others mumble constantly?
- Turn up the TV louder than others prefer.
- Avoid phone calls because they're hard to follow.
- Feel drained after social events or meetings?
- Struggle to hear your partner from another room?
- Nod and smile even when you're not sure what was said?

If you answered "yes" to two or more questions, it's time for a hearing screening.

Appendix B

Starting the Conversation with a Loved One

Are you unsure how to discuss hearing healthcare with a loved one? Try this:

What NOT to say:

- *"You really need hearing aids."*
- *"You're not listening to me!"*
- *"You're going deaf."*

Try this instead:

- *"I've noticed it's harder to talk like we used to. Have you noticed that too?"*
- *"I miss having conversations with you without repeating everything."*
- *"I read this book and it made me realize how much hearing affects everything. Want to check it out with me?"*

Keep it compassionate, not corrective. Hearing loss is emotional and it deserves empathy.

Appendix C

Frequently Asked Questions

Q: Will hearing aids make everything sound normal again?

A: Not overnight. But with the right settings and a little time, most people adapt and hear better than they have in years.

Q: What if I already have memory issues? Is it too late?

A: No. Treating hearing loss may slow further cognitive decline, even in people with mild dementia.

Q: I've heard hearing aids are expensive. Are there other options?

A: Yes. Hearing aids now come in a range of prices and technology levels to fit most budgets. Over-the-counter (OTC) options are available for mild to moderate hearing loss, but for the best results, seeing a hearing care provider is key. Proper fit, personalized settings, and follow-up care make all the difference in long-term success.

Q: I've had tinnitus for years—can hearing aids still help?

A: Often, yes. Especially if it's related to hearing loss. Many hearing aids offer tinnitus-masking features too.

Q: How do I find a provider I can trust?

A: Look for one who listens first, explains clearly, and offers follow-up care, not just a sales pitch.

Q: What if I tried hearing aids before and didn't like them?

A: Technology has improved dramatically in recent years. If they didn't work for you then, it doesn't mean they won't now. It's also important to find the right provider to help you fine-tune the fit and sound.

Q: Do I really need two hearing aids if only one ear seems worse?

A: In most cases, yes. Hearing is a two-ear process. Wearing aids in both ears helps with balance, clarity, and understanding speech—especially in noisy places.

Q: Will people notice I'm wearing hearing aids?

A: Probably not. Many modern hearing aids are nearly invisible. What they will notice is that you're more engaged, confident, and connected.

Q: How long does it take to get used to hearing aids?

A: Everyone's timeline is different, but most people adjust within a few weeks. The key is consistent use, a good fit, and support from a provider who can make needed adjustments along the way.

Appendix D

Hearing Appointment Checklist

What to bring. What to ask. What to expect.

Your Appointment Checklist:

- Write down your top questions or concerns
- Be aware of specific situations where you struggle to hear (restaurants, phone, TV, etc.)
- Can a family member or friend come with you? (optional but helpful)
- Gather a list of medications and medical history
- Schedule time for a full hearing evaluation and discussion (plan for 60–90 minutes)
- Insurance card (if applicable)
- Plan to bring your current hearing aids (if you have them)

Questions to Ask During the Visit

- What type of hearing loss do I have?
- How is it affecting my brain, memory, or mood?
- Would hearing aids help me?
- Are there non-device options I should know about?
- What will the adjustment process be like?

- Can you help with tinnitus or ringing in the ears?
- What happens if I do nothing?

What to Expect

- A conversation about your concerns
- A full hearing evaluation (not just a quick screening)
- Explanation of your results in plain language
- Time to ask questions
- Recommendations based on your lifestyle and goals
- A follow-up plan, if you're not ready to move forward today

After the Appointment

- You should understand your hearing test results
- You I know what next steps were recommended
- You feel comfortable reaching out with more questions
- You have scheduled a follow-up appointment if needed

Pro Tip: Bring a notebook or use your phone to jot down anything you want to remember.

Suggested Reading & Support Resources

This section includes helpful organizations, research summaries, and additional information related to hearing loss, tinnitus, mental health, and cognitive wellness. These resources were selected to support readers who want to learn more, seek community, or explore science in greater depth.

Understanding Hearing Loss & Brain Health

Johns Hopkins School of Medicine – Dr. Frank Lin
Research from Dr. Lin and his team explores the links between hearing loss and cognitive decline, including studies like the ACHIEVE trial (2023).
https://www.johnshopkinsmedicine.org

The ACHIEVE Study (2023)
A major randomized controlled trial showing that treating hearing loss can help slow cognitive decline in older adults.
Deal et al., The Lancet, 2023

American Journal of Public Health (2016)
Goman & Lin: Prevalence of hearing loss and its broader societal impact.
https://doi.org/10.2105/AJPH.2016.303299

Tinnitus Support & Management

American Tinnitus Association (ATA)

A trusted source for tinnitus research, coping tools, sound therapy options, and current news.

https://www.ata.org

Tinnitus Retraining Therapy – Jastreboff Model

Details the neurophysiological model explaining how tinnitus is managed through sound therapy and counseling.

Mental Health & Hearing Loss

JAMA Otolaryngology – Hearing Aids and Depression Study (2020)

Choi et al.: Found reduced depressive symptoms among older adults using hearing aids or cochlear implants.

https://doi.org/10.1001/jamaoto.2020.0480

The National Council on Aging (NCOA)

Offers summaries of landmark surveys on how untreated hearing loss affects emotional well-being.

https://www.ncoa.org

Mener et al. (2013), Journal of the American Geriatrics Society

Findings on hearing loss and increased risk of depression

in older adults.

https://www.ncbi.nlm.nih.gov/pmc/articles/PMC9884987

Advocacy & Education

Hearing Loss Association of America (HLAA)
Education, support networks, and advocacy for individuals with hearing loss.

https://www.hearingloss.org

National Institute on Deafness and Other Communication (NIDCD)
Government-backed research and statistics on hearing, balance, tinnitus, and communication disorders.

https://www.nidcd.nih.gov

Better Hearing Institute (BHI)
Dedicated to public awareness about hearing loss and the benefits of treatment.

https://www.betterhearing.org

Reminder: If you're facing hearing loss, tinnitus, or related mental health challenges, help is available. These resources can guide you toward the support and answers you need to take the next step.

References

American Tinnitus Association. (n.d.). *Understanding the facts.* https://www.ata.org

Arlinger, S. (2003). Negative consequences of uncorrected hearing loss–a review. *International Journal of Audiology, 42*(Suppl 2), 17–20. https://doi.org/10.3109/14992020309074639

Choi, J. S., Betz, J., Li, L., Reed, N. S., Lin, F. R., & Deal, J. A. (2020). Association of using hearing aids or cochlear implants with changes in depressive symptoms in older adults. *JAMA Otolaryngology–Head & Neck Surgery, 146*(7), 630–638. https://doi.org/10.1001/jamaoto.2020.0480

Deal, J. A., Albert, M. S., Arnold, M., Bangdiwala, S. I., Chisolm, T., Davis, S., ... & Lin, F. R. (2023). Hearing intervention versus health education control to reduce cognitive decline in older adults with hearing loss in the USA (ACHIEVE): A multicentre, randomized controlled trial. *The Lancet, 402*(10405), 1873–1882. https://doi.org/10.1016/S0140-6736(23)01544-2

Goman, A. M., & Lin, F. R. (2016). Prevalence of hearing loss by severity in the United States. *American Journal of Public Health, 106*(10), 1820–1822. https://doi.org/10.2105/AJPH.2016.303299

Hearing Loss Association of America. (n.d.). *Facts about hearing loss.* https://www.hearingloss.org

Jensen, J. H., Steel, Z., & Lind, C. (2019). The impact of hearing loss on mental health: A systematic review. *International Journal of Audiology, 58*(10), 613–620. https://doi.org/10.1080/14992027.2019.1626636

Lin, F. R., & Albert, M. (2014). Hearing loss and dementia – who is listening? *Aging & Mental Health, 18*(6), 671–673. https://doi.org/10.1080/13607863.2014.915924

Lin, F. R., Yaffe, K., Xia, J., Xue, Q. L., Harris, T. B., Purchase-Helzner, E., ... & Simonsick, E. M. (2013). Hearing loss and cognitive decline in older adults. *JAMA Internal Medicine, 173*(4), 293–299. https://doi.org/10.1001/jamainternmed.2013.1868

Livingston, G., Huntley, J., Sommerlad, A., Ames, D., Ballard, C., Banerjee, S., ... & Mukadam, N. (2020). Dementia prevention, intervention, and care: 2020 report of the Lancet Commission. *The Lancet, 396*(10248), 413–446. https://doi.org/10.1016/S0140-6736(20)30367-6

Mener, D. J., Betz, J., Genther, D. J., Chen, D., & Lin, F. R. (2013). Hearing loss and depression in older adults. *Journal of the American Geriatrics Society, 61*(9), 1627–1629. https://www.ncbi.nlm.nih.gov/pmc/articles/PMC9884987

National Council on Aging. (1999). *The consequences of untreated hearing loss in older persons.* https://www.ncoa.org/article/can-hearing-loss-affect-mental-health-in-older-adults

National Institute on Deafness and Other Communication Disorders. (n.d.). *Quick statistics about hearing.* https://www.nidcd.nih.gov/health/statistics/quick-statistics-hearing

Pronk, M., Deeg, D. J., Smits, C., Twisk, J. W., van Tilburg, T. G., & Kramer, S. E. (2014). Hearing loss and cognitive decline in older adults: The impact of hearing aid use. *The Journals of Gerontology: Series B, 69*(3), 425–432. https://pubmed.ncbi.nlm.nih.gov/38925313

Sharma, A. (n.d.). *Neuroplasticity in hearing loss and auditory deprivation.* American Geriatrics Society. (Referenced in a conference presentation; full paper unavailable for public link.)

Shukla, A., Harper, M., Pedersen, E., Goman, A., Suen, J. J., Price, C., & Lin, F. R. (2020). Hearing loss, loneliness, and social isolation: A systematic review. *Otolaryngology–Head and Neck Surgery, 162*(5), 622–633. https://doi.org/10.1177/0194599820910377

U.S. Department of Veterans Affairs. (2019). *Hearing loss, tinnitus, and mental health risks among U.S. veterans.* (Summary publication).

Zuelke, A. E., et al. (2019). Suicide ideation among adults with hearing loss: United States, 2007–2014. *JAMA Otolaryngology–Head & Neck Surgery, 145*(7), 608–610.

Prescott Hearing Center and the Author

At Prescott Hearing Center, we believe better hearing is about more than just sound. It's about connection, confidence, and quality of life.

My name is Doug Dunker, and I've spent over 25 years helping people navigate the emotional and practical challenges of hearing loss. I've seen firsthand how the right support can restore not only hearing, but relationships, independence, and peace of mind. This book was written to shed light on what so many people struggle with in silence and to offer a path forward.

Prescott Hearing Center was built on a simple belief: care should be personal, compassionate, and comprehensive. Whether it's hearing loss, tinnitus, or just the sense that something is "off," our team is here to listen, support, and help you rediscover what connections really sound like.

We don't just fit hearing aids, we walk with people through a process of real, lasting improvement. We are honored to be part of that journey with you.

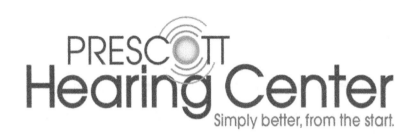

Prescott Hearing Center was established with the goal of providing quality and affordable hearing solutions to the community of Prescott, and the Quad-City area in Yavapai County, Arizona.

Schedule An Appt Now
☎ (928) 899-8104

PrescottHearing.com

Prescott Hearing Center Locations

3108 Clearwater Dr. Suite B2
Prescott, AZ 86305

7762 E. Florentine Rd. Suite D
Prescott Valley, AZ 86314